MCQs IN OTOLOGY FOR UNDEGRADUATE MEDICAL STUDENTS

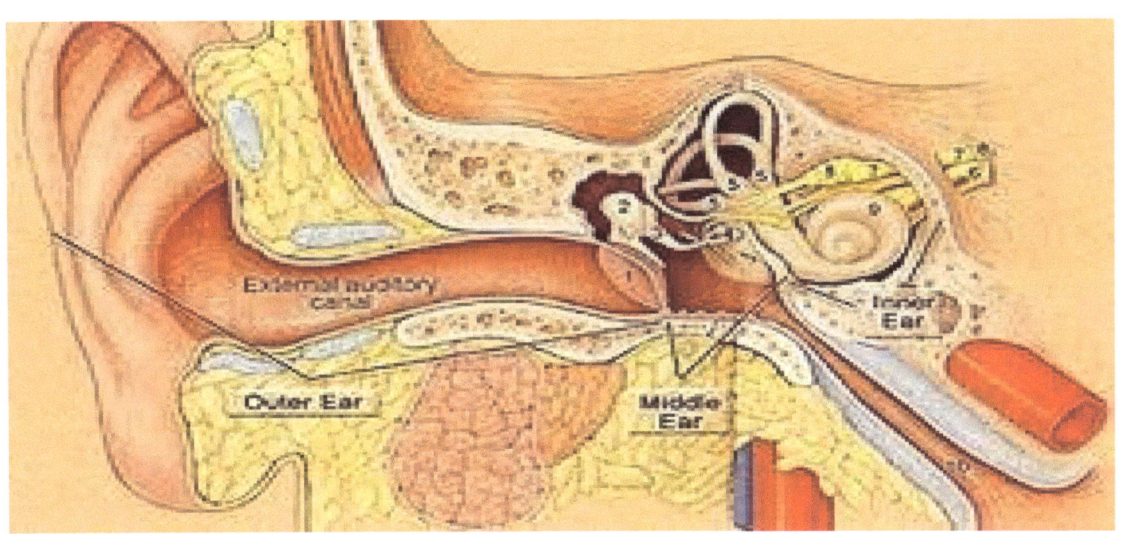

MEHDEE HASSAN & AUNG K SOE

UniKL RCMP

MCQs IN OTOLOGY FOR UNDERGRADUATE MEDICAL STUDENTS

Mehdee Hassan MBBS, DLO, MS (ENT)

Senior Lecturer (ENT)

University Kuala Lumpur Royal College of Medicine Perak (UniKL RCMP)

Aung K Soe MBBS, M.Med.Sc (Otorhinolaryngology)

Senior Lecturer (ENT)

University Kuala Lumpur Royal College of Medicine Perak (UniKL RCMP)

PREFACE

This book is the culmination of more than 10 years of experience in otorhinolaryngology. We wish to express our gratitude to all our mentors, teachers and colleagues whose constant encouragement and support has resulted in this book. We specially would like to thank Professor Dr Osman Ali, Dean (Faculty of Medicine, UniKL RCMP), Professor Dato' Dr Subramaniam Muniandy, Head of Surgery based Department (UniKL RCMP) and Dr Sandheep Sugathan, Senior Lecturer (UniKL RCMP) for all their support in getting this book published.

We are also thankful to all our students, who have constantly challenged us with their questions. Lastly, we are deeply indebted to our beloved family members for the time taken from them in preparing this book.

We sincerely hope that this book helps you to your examination and wish you all the best in your medical career!

Mehdee Hassan & Aung K Soe   December 2015

SECTION A

1. A 65-year-old lady presented with a painless, smelly discharge from her right ear, which developed over a few months. Upon further inquiry she claims that she now has to use the telephone on her left ear as she finds it difficult to hear on the right. What is the most likely diagnosis?
    a. Otitis externa
    b. Otitis media
    c. Squamous cell carcinoma
    d. Cholesteatoma
    e. Presbyacusis

2. Which ONE of the following is the commonest causative organism in necrotising otitis externa?
    a. Pseudomonas aeruginosa
    b. Klebsiella
    c. Aspergillus niger
    d. Clostridium species
    e. Staphylococcus aureus

3. Type C tympanogram is consistent with
    a. Secretory otitis media
    b. Otosclerosis
    c. Eustachian tube dysfunction
    d. Ossicular discontinuity.

4. The expected type of tympanogram in secretory otitis media is
    a. Type B
    b. Type C
    c. Type As
    d. Type Ad

5. In a 40-year-old female patient with left hearing loss, Rinne test is negative on the left side and tympanogram is Type As, your diagnosis is
    a. Left secretory otitis media.
    b. Left otosclerosis.
    c. Left tympanosclerosis
    d. All are true

6. A 5-year-old child has persistent serous effusions in both ears for 6 months after a routine acute infection. He has a 40-dB conductive hearing loss in both ears and has been having trouble in school. What would be the BEST treatment for this child?
    a. Observe the child for another 3 months
    b. Prescribe amoxicillin for 10 days

c. Recommend hearing aids
   d. Place ventilating tubes
   e. Prescribe prophylactic antibiotics for 3 months

7. By central drum perforation we mean:
   a. Perforation at the central part of the drum
   b. A perforation in the pars tensa which is surrounded by a rim of tympanic membrane
   c. A perforation of the pars flaccida
   d. A perforation in the pars tensa which is not surrounded by a rim of tympanic membrane

8. A 30-year-old patient with recurrent attacks of vertigo, hearing loss and tinnitus associated with nausea and vomiting has
   a. Benign paroxysmal positional vertigo
   b. Vestibular neuronitis.
   c. Meniere's disease
   d. Acoustic neuroma.

9. The combination of unilateral otorrhoea, severe facial pain and diplopia is known as
   a. Pierre Robin syndrome
   b. Gradenigo's syndrome
   c. Kartagener's syndrome
   d. Ramsay Hunt syndrome

10. Uncontrolled diabetes in elderly patient may predispose to
   a. Cholesteatoma
   b. Malignant otitis externa
   c. Presbyacusis
   d. Vestibular neuronitis

11. Diplopia on looking to the left side in a patient with a history of bilateral chronic suppurative otitis media is likely due to
   a. Right petrositis
   b. Left lateral sinus thrombophlebitis.
   c. Right petrositis affecting the abducent nerve
   d. Left petrositis affecting the abducent nerve

12. Cholesteatoma causes fistula commonly in:
   a. Promontory
   b. Lateral semicircular canal
   c. Posterior semicircular canal
   d. Stapes footplate

13. In Gradenigo syndrome diplopia is due to inflammation of the following cranial nerve
   a. IV nerve
   b. V nerve
   c. III Nerve
   d. VI nerve

14. **In traumatic rupture of the drum, which of the following is true:**
    a. The main treatment is conservative.
    b. Local ear drops are highly indicated.
    c. It usually heals spontaneously within 3 months.
    d. Myringoplasty is the first line of treatment.

15. **In upper motor neurone facial paralysis**
    a. The upper part of the face is spared
    b. The lower part of the face is spared
    c. Both upper half and lower half are paralyzed
    d. Hypotonia of facial muscles is characteristic of this type.

16. **In lower motor neurone facial paralysis with intact taste sensation at the anterior 2/3 of the tongue, the level of the lesion is**
    a. In the internal auditory canal
    b. In the horizontal tympanic part
    c. In the vertical part above the stapes
    d. In the stylomastoid foramen

17. **The early symptom of Bell's palsy is:**
    a. Dropping of angle of the affected side.
    b. Obliteration of the angle of the mouth.
    c. Pain of acute onset behind the ear.
    d. Inability to close the eye.

18. **A patient with facial nerve paralysis suffers intolerance of loud sound due to denervation of which muscle**
    a. Posterior belly of digastric
    b. Tensor tympani
    c. Stapedius muscle
    d. All of the above.

19. **The best investigation for diagnosis of vestibular schwannoma is**
    a. CT scan.
    b. MRI
    c. ABR
    d. Pure tone audiogram

20. **In management of auricular hematoma,**
    a. Aspiration of blood is only needed
    b. Systemic antibiotic is sufficient
    c. Evacuation of blood followed by pressure bandage is the proper management
    d. No treatment is needed because it will resolve spontaneously.

21. **By modified radical mastoidectomy we mean**
    a. Removal of mastoid air cells and all middle ear contents
    b. Removal of diseased mastoid air cells

c. Removal of mastoid air cells and all middle ear contents with preservation of healthy remnants of tympanic membrane and ossicles
  d. None of the above.

22. **The most common complication of myringotomy operation is**
    a. Injury of facial nerve.
    b. Dislocation of the incus
    c. Injury of the jugular bulb
    d. Residual perforation

23. **The commonest cause of unilateral sensorineural hearing loss is**
    a. Ototoxic poisoning.
    b. Measles
    c. Mumps.
    d. Rh incompatibility
    e. Syphilis.

24. **Fluctuant SNHL usually occurs in:**
    a. Presbyacusis
    b. Meniere's disease.
    c. Otosclerosis.
    d. All of the above.

25. **In a patient suffering from sudden severe vertigo lasting for 2 days which resolves spontaneously, but hearing is normal, the diagnosis is likely**
    a. Meniere's disease
    b. Vestibular neuronitis
    c. Labyrinthitis
    d. Vestibular schwannoma

26. **The commonest cause of vertigo is**
    a. Meniere's disease
    b. Labyrinthitis
    c. Benign paroxysmal positional vertigo
    d. Ototoxicity

27. **Mixed hearing loss may be caused by one of the following:**
    a. Otosclerosis.
    b. Meniere's disease.
    c. Ear wax.
    d. Acoustic neuroma.

28. **Etiology for pulsatile tinnitus includes the followings except:**
    a. Arteriovenous malformation of neck.
    b. Otosclerosis.
    c. Glomus jugulare tumors.
    d. Hyperthyroidism.

29. **Slowly progressive conductive deafness in middle aged female with normal drum & Eustachian tube function is most probably due to:**
   a. Otitis media with effusion.
   b. Otosclerosis.
   c. Malingering.
   d. Tympanosclerosis.

30. **The IX, X and XI cranial nerves may be involved in all of the following except**
   a. Acoustic neuroma
   b. Transverse temporal bone fracture.
   c. Malignant otitis externa
   d. Squamous cell carcinoma of the middle ear.

31. **The following have an ototoxic effect except**
   a. Gentamycin
   b. Furosemide
   c. Streptomycin
   d. Amoxicillin
   e. Quinine.

32. **Referred otalgia from pyriform sinus cancer is through:**
   a. IX cranial nerve
   b. X cranial nerve
   c. XII cranial nerve
   d. VII cranial nerve

33. **The maximum output of a 512 tuning fork is:**
a. 50 dB
b. 60 dB
c. 70 dB
d. 80 dB
e. 90 dB.

34. **Griesinger's sign is:**
a. Edema & tenderness over the posterior border of the mastoid process.
b. Unilateral pulsating otorrhoea.
c. Vertigo & nystagmus on increasing the pressure of the EAC.
d. Tenderness on the tip of mastoid bone.

35. **The fluids presents in secretory otitis media is:**
a. Mucopurulent.
b. Serosanguinous.
c. Exudates. d. Transudates.
e. Mixture of exudates & transudates.

36. **The discharge in case of cholesteatoma is:**
a. Copious purulent.
b. Copious offensive.
c. Scanty offensive.

d. Thick scanty creamy.

37. The following is true about pure tone audiometry EXCEPT:
a. It gives the amount of the hearing loss in dB.
b. It gives the type of deafness.
c. It helps in hearing aid selection.
d. It helps in follow up of the case.
e. It measures the sound emitted from the cochlea.

38. Bell's palsy is LMNL at the level of:
a. Geniculate ganglion.
b. Internal facial auditory meatus.
c. Stylomastoid foramen.
d. Cerebellopontine angle.

39. The cause of Bell's palsy may be one of the following EXCEPT:
a. Vascular ischemia.
b. Virus infection.
c. Bacterial infection.
d. Auto immune.

40. Longitudinal fracture of the temporal bone may be associated with all of the following EXCEPT:
a. LMNL facial palsy.
b. Traumatic perforation of the tympanic membrane.
c. Conductive hearing loss. d. Profound hearing loss.

41. ABR "Auditory Brain stem Response" is used in:
a. Test of hearing in malingering.
b. Test of hearing in retrocochlear lesion.
c. Detection of acoustic neuroma.
d. All of the above.

42. The following are the manifestations of temporal lobe abscess EXCEPT:
a. Hemiparesis.
b. Aphasia.
c. Convulsive fits.
d. Vertigo.

43. The most accurate diagnostic test to detect degeneration of the facial nerve:
a. Nerve excitability test.
b. Electromyography.
c. Electroneurography.
d. Stapedial reflex.

44. Unilateral hearing loss with pulsating tinnitus is suggestive of:
a. Otosclerosis.
b. Extradural abscess complicating CSOM.
c. Glomus tumor.
d. Acoustic neuroma.

45. A case of ear infection followed by headache, blurring of vision & vomiting is suggestive of:
a. Mastoiditis.
b. Petrositis.
c. Labyrinthitis.
d. Brain abscess.

46. Mixed hearing loss may be caused by one of the following:
a. Otosclerosis.
b. Meniere's disease.
c. Ear wax.
d. Acoustic neuroma.

47. The triad of ear discharge, retro-orbital pain & 6th nerve paralysis is due to:
a. Mastoiditis.
b. Labyrinthitis.
c. Apical petrositis.
d. Lateral sinus thrombosis.

48. Fever, headache, vomiting & neck rigidity in a patient with cholesteatoma is an indication of:
a. Lumbar puncture.
b. CT scan.
c. Fundus examination,
d. All of the above.

49. Fever & rigor developing in a case of cholesteatoma is suggestive of:
a. Cerebellar abscess.
b. Acute mastoiditis.
c. Lateral sinus thrombosis.
d. Labyrinthitis.

50. Equilibrium during angular "rotational" movement is the function of:
a. The utricle.
b. The saccule.
c. The cochlea.
d. The semicircular canal.

51. A 5-year-old child has persistent serous effusions in both ears for 6 months after a routine acute infection. He has a 40-dB conductive hearing loss in both ears and has been having trouble in school. What would be the BEST treatment for this child?
a. Observe the child for another 3 months
b. Prescribe amoxicillin for 10 days
c. Recommend hearing aids
d. Place ventilating tubes
e. Prescribe prophylactic antibiotics for 3 months

52. The concept that the facial nerve supplies the auricle is related to:
a. Ramsay-Hunt syndrome.

b. Jugular foramen syndrome.
c. Horner's syndrome.
d. Bell's palsy.

53. Topognostic test is used in the assessment of facial paralysis include all the following EXCEPT:
a. Schirmer test.
b. Stapedial reflex.
c. Electroneurography.
d. Gustatory test.

54. A child with an attic drum perforation who developed nausea, projectile vomiting and fever of 40 degree is suspicious to have got
a. Otogenic meningitis
b. Otogenic labyrinthitis
c. Petrositis
d. Mastoiditis

55. A large near total perforation following acute necrotizing otitis media must be followed up for fear of
a. Recurrent middle ear infection.
b. Secondary acquired cholesteatoma.
c. Retraction pocket.
d. Tympanosclerosis.

56. Treatment of acute otitis media must continue until
a. Vomiting stops
b. Fever becomes normal
c. Hearing becomes normal
d. Pain is relieved.

57. An early and diagnostic sign of mastoiditis is:
a. Reservoir sign.
b. Sagging of the postero-superior part of the bony canal.
c. Perforated tympanic membrane.
d. Post-auricular mastoid abscess.

58. A patient with long standing left otorrhea presented with persistent left temporal headache, the diagnosis may be
a. Migraine.
b. Mastoiditis
c. Extradural abscess.
d. Meningitis.

59. The tympanic membrane perforation in acute otitis media is
a. Central in the pars tensa
b. Marginal in the pars tensa
c. Small in the pars flaccida
d. None of the above.

60. In Injury of the facial nerve at the horizontal tympanic part
a. The facial muscles are paralyzed at the opposite side
b. Lacrimation is affected at the same side
c. Salivation is affected at the same side
d. All of the above.

61. The test of hearing in infants is:
a. Rinne test.
b. Weber test.
c. Pure tone audiometry.
d. ABR (Auditory Brain stem Response).

62. In a 50 years old patient presenting with right hearing loss and tinnitus of one month duration. His pure tone audiogram showed right sensorineural hearing loss. Which of the following is not true:
a. Presbyacusis is suspected
b. Nothing is done and annual follow up is only needed.
c. Acoustic neuroma is suspected.
d. MRI is the best investigation to uncover the diagnosis.
e. a and b
f. c and d

63. Before myringoplasty in a 30 years old patient, the following is required
a. Audiogram
b. Ensure dry perforation
c. Treatment of any underlying nasal or paranasal sinus infection
d. All of the above
e. None of the above

64. By modified radical mastoidectomy we mean
a. Removal of mastoid air cells and all middle ear contents
b. Removal of diseased mastoid air cells
c. Removal of mastoid air cells and all middle ear contents with preservation of healthy remnants of tympanic membrane and ossicles
d. None of the above.

65. The aim of radical mastoidectomy is:
a. To make the ear safe.
b. To preserve hearing.
c. Reconstruct the ossicles.
d. Reconstruct the tympanic membrane

66. In myringotomy operation the posterosuperior quadrant of the tympanic membrane must be avoided
a. To avoid injury of dehiscent jugular bulb.
b. To avoid injury of the ossicles.
c. None of the above

67. The first line of treatment in a child who develops lower motor neurone facial paralysis after acute otitis media is

a. Antibiotics and corticosteroids.
b. Decompression of facial nerve.
c. Exploration of facial nerve
d. Myringotomy

68. Cochlear implant is indicated in patients having
a. Bilateral conductive hearing loss
b. Bilateral sensorineural hearing loss
c. Bilateral total hearing loss who cannot gain benefit from hearing aids.
d. All of the above.

69. Which of the following is associated with objective tinnitus?
a. Ménière's disease.
b. Ear wax impaction.
c. Acoustic neuroma.
d. Palatal myoclonus.
e. Middle ear effusion

70. In a patient suffering from sudden severe vertigo lasting for 2 days which resolves spontaneously, but hearing is normal, the diagnosis is likely
a. Meniere's disease
b. Vestibular neuronitis
c. Labyrinthitis
d. Vestibular schwannoma

71. In Paracusis Willisii
a. The patient hears better in quiet places.
b. The patient hears better in noisy places.
c. The patient has sensorineural hearing loss.
d. The patient cannot tolerate loud sound.

72. Which of the following drugs are known to cause tinnitus?
a. Salicylates.
b. Loop Diuretics.
c. Aminoglycosides.
d. NSAID.
e. All of the above

73. A 35 years old female patient presented with right tinnitus 1 year ago followed by slowly progressive right hearing loss after 6 months. Otoscopic examination was completely normal. Pure tone audiometry reveals right high frequency sensorineural hearing loss. Speech discrimination test and auditory brain stem response (ABR) showed abnormal findings. The most valuable investigation to detect an early lesion would be:
a. MRI of the IAC.
b. MRI of the brain and IAC.
c. CT of the brain and IAC.
d. Contrast CT of the IAC.
e. PET of the IAC

74. Endolymph is formed in:

a. Utricle.
b. Endolymphatic sac.
c. Scala media.
d. Scala tympani.
e. Saccule.

75. The cough response caused while cleaning the ear canal is mediated by stimulation of:
a. The 5th cranial nerve.
b. Innervation of external ear canal by C_1 and C_2.
c. The 10th cranial nerve.
d. Branches of the 7th cranial nerve.

76. A 38-year-old gentleman reported of decreased hearing in the right ear for the last two years. On testing with a 512-Hz tuning fork, the Rinne's test was negative on the right ear and positive on the left. With the Weber's test the tone was perceived louder in the left ear. The patient most likely had:
a. Right conductive hearing loss.
b. Right sensorineural hearing loss.
c. Left sensorineural hearing loss.
d. Left conductive hearing loss.

77. Referred otalgia is frequently encountered in an otolaryngology practice. Referred pain from a base of tongue lesion involves the:
   a. Gasserian ganglion
   b. Petrosal ganglion
   c. Sphenopalatine ganglion
   d. Otic ganglion
   e. Nodose ganglion.

78. The muscles involved in the function of the eustachian tube include all of the following EXCEPT:
   a. Tensor tympani
   b. Tensor palati
   c. Levator palati
   d. Salpingopharyngeus
   e. Salpingopalatus.

79. Cupulolithiasis is an entity believed to be due to:
   a. Dislodgement of the statoconia of the saccule to the horizontal canal
   b. Dislodgement of the statoconia of the saccule to the posterior canal
   c. Dislodgement of the statoconia of the utricle to the horizontal canal
   d. Dislodgement of the statoconia of the utricle to the posterior canal
   e. Free-floating statoconia in all three semicircular canals.

80. The membranous labyrinth is derived from:
   a. Ectoderm
   b. Mesoderm
   c. Entoderm
   d. Ectoderm and mesoderm

81. The most accurate noninvasive test for acoustic neuroma diagnosis is:
   a. Computerized cranial tomography
   b. Auditory brain stem responses
   c. The crossed acoustic reflex
   d. Temporal bone polytomography
   e. Electronystagmography.

82. Unilateral hearing loss with pulsating tinnitus is suggestive of:
a. Otosclerosis.
b. Extradural abscess complicating CSOM.
c. Glomus tumor.
d. Acoustic neuroma.

83. The earliest symptom in a case with cholesteatoma that indicates intracranial complication is:
a. Persistent headache.
b. Facial palsy.
c. SNHL.
d. Squint.

84. The most common cause of otitis media with effusion is:
a. Inadequate treatment of acute otitis media.
b. Nasopharyngeal neoplasm.
c. Allergy.
d. Otitic barotraumas.

85. A 25-year-old woman suffering from bilateral hearing loss for 6 years which become profound with pregnancy. On tympanogram which of the following curve is obtained?
a. A_D
b. A_S
c. A
d. B

86. A 7-year-old child developed acute otitis media. He was treated with antibiotics for 10 days. His pain and fever subsided completely but still had conductive hearing loss. The next line of treatment is:
a. To give another course of different antibiotic.
b. To do a myringotomy and culture the middle ear fluid.
c. To do a myringotomy and insert a grommet.
d. To wait and watch for 3 months for fluid to drain spontaneously.

87. Which of the following is not a typical feature of Ménière's disease?
a. Sensorineural hearing loss.
b. Pulsatile tinnitus.
c. Vertigo.
Fluctuating hearing loss.

88. Which of the following is not a typical feature of malignant otitis externa?
a. Caused by *Pseudomonas aeruginosa*.
b. Patients are usually elderly.

c. Mitotic figures are high.
d. Patients are immunocompromised.

89. Which of the following is true regarding facial nerve palsy associated with temporal bone fracture?
a. Common with longitudinal fracture.
b. Common with transverse fracture.
c. Always associated with CSF otorrhoea.
d. Facial nerve injury is always complete.

90. Which is the investigation of choice in assessing hearing loss in neonates?
a. Impedance audiometry.
b. Brainstem evoked response audiometry.
c. Free field audiometry.
d. Behavioural audiometry.

91. Which of the following conditions causes the maximum hearing loss?
a. Ossicular disruption with intact tympanic membrane.
b. Disruption of malleus and incus as well as tympanic membrane.
c. Partial fixation of stapes footplate.
d. Otitis media with effusion.

92. Otoacoustic emissions are produced by:
a. Inner hair cells.
b. Outer hair cells.
c. Basilar membrane.
d. Auditory nerve.

93. Speech frequencies are:
a. 125 250 500 Hz.
b. 250 500 1000 Hz.
c. 500 1000 2000 Hz.
d. 1000 2000 4000 Hz.

94. Caloric test determines the function of:
a. Superior semicircular canal.
b. Lateral semicircular canal.
c. Posterior semicircular canal.
d. Utricle.

95. In episodic positional vertigo, which of the following tests is used?
a. Caloric test.
b. Dix-Hallpike manoeuvre.
c. Rotation test.
d. Electronystagmography.

96. All of the following drugs are used to treat otomycosis except:
a. 2% salicylic acid.
b. 5% soda-bicarb.
c. 1% gentian violet.

d. Clotrimazole.

97. Treatment of dry traumatic rupture of tympanic membrane is:
a. Antibiotic ear drop.
b. Myringoplasty.
c. Protection of ear against water.
d. Ear pack soaked with antibiotic.

98. A 5-year-old boy has been diagnosed to have posterosuperior retraction pocket with cholesteatoma. All would constitute part of management except:
a. Audiometry.
b. Mastoid exploration.
c. Tympanoplasty.
d. Myringoplasty.

99. A 10-year-old boy presented with torticollis, a tender swelling behind the angle of mandible and fever. He had history of ear discharge for the past 6 years. Examination of the ear showed purulent discharge and granulations in the ear canal. Most probable diagnosis is:
a. Acute lymphadenitis secondary to otitis externa.
b. Masked mastoiditis.
c. Bezold's abscess.
d. Parotitis.

100. Longstanding case of otitis media with effusion can develop all of the following complications except:
a. Retraction pocket.
b. Cholesteatoma.
c. Ossicular fixation.
d. Middle ear atelectasis.
e. Cholesterol granuloma.

101. All of the following statements are true about Carhart's notch except:
a. It is a sensorineural hearing loss.
b. Maximum loss is centred at 2 kHz.
c. Seen only in stapes fixation.
d. Cannot be reversed.

102. Condition in which loud sounds produce giddiness is called:
a. Paracusis Willisii.
b. Hennebert's sign.
c. Tullio phenomenon.
d. Otolithic crisis of Tumarkin.

103. A 31-year-old female patient complained of bilateral hearing impairment for the past 5 years. On examination, tympanic membrane was normal, and audiogram showed a bilateral conductive loss. Impedance audiometry showed As type of curve and absent acoustic reflex. All constitutes part of treatment except:
a. Hearing aid.
b. Stapedectomy.

c. Sodium fluoride.
d. Gentamicin therapy.

104. In acoustic neuroma, cranial nerve to be involved earliest is:
a. V.
b. VII.
c. X.
d. IX.

105. The most common cause of peripheral episodic vertigo is:
a. Meniere's disease.
b. Acoustic neuroma.
c. Benign paroxysmal positional vertigo.
d. Vascular occlusion of labyrinthine artery.

106. All are true about benign paroxysmal positional vertigo except:
a. More often occurs after 40 years of age.
b. Males are affected more than female.
c. Follows an attack of vestibular neuronitis.
d. Head trauma or ear surgery predisposes to BPPV.

107. With the tuning fork of 512 Hz, Weber test is lateralised to the right ear. It denotes:
a. Conductive hearing loss on the right ear and normal on the left.
b. Normal right ear but sensorineural hearing loss on the left.
c. Conductive hearing loss on the left ear with normal right ear.
d. Both a and b.

108. Which of the following statements is incorrect about Acoustic neuroma?
a. Vertigo is severe and often precedes hearing loss.
b. Difficulty in understanding speech is out of proportion to hearing loss.
c. Facial palsy is a late feature.
d. Unilateral tinnitus and sensorineural hearing loss is the earliest symptom.

109. High frequency sensorineural hearing loss after head injury is most often caused by:
a. Injury to the auditory nerve.
b. Fracture of the bony cochlea.
c. Concussion of the labyrinth.
d. The brain haemorrhage.

110. A hearing aid consists of the following components except:
a. Microphone.
b. Amplifier.
c. Receiver.
d. speech processor.

111. All of the following drugs are ototoxic except:
a. Chloroquine.
b. Cotrimoxazole.
c. Cisplatin.
d. Frusemide.

112. **Adenoidectomy is indicated in all of the following conditions except:**
a. Otitis media with effusion.
b. Nasal obstruction due to adenoid hyperplasia.
c. Recurrent otitis media in children.
d. Allergic rhinitis in children.

113. **In Ramsay-Hunt syndrome, which of the following ganglia does herpes zoster involve?**
a. Scarpa's ganglion.
b. Spiral ganglion.
c. Geniculate ganglion.
d. Stellate ganglion.

114. **Hypaesthesia of the posterior meatal wall is seen in:**
a. Vestibular Schwannoma.
b. Glomus tympanicum.
c. Carcinoma of the middle ear.
d. Lateral sinus thrombosis.

115. **An elderly man had longstanding ear discharge; and now presented with facial palsy, ear pain which was worse at night and a friable polyp in the ear with tendency to bleed. The likely diagnosis is:**
a. CSOM with polyp.
b. Malignant otitis externa.
c. Carcinoma of middle ear.
d. Glomus tumour.

116. **All are true about longitudinal fracture of temporal bone except:**
a. Longitudinal fractures occur less commonly than transverse fractures.
b. Less chances of facial palsy.
c. Occurs due to a blow from the side.
d. Causes conductive hearing loss.

117. **Recurrent facial paralysis is seen in all except:**
a. Acoustic neuroma.
b. Diabetes.
c. Sarcoidosis.
d. Cholesteatoma

118. **Smallest segment of facial nerve is:**
a. Intracanalicular.
b. Labyrinthine.
c. Tympanic.
d. Mastoid.
e. Parotid segment before its division.

119. **Following landmarks are useful in locating the facial nerve except:**
a. Nerve passes above the oval window.
b. Nerve courses above the horizontal canal.

c. Nerve exits anterior to digastric ridge.
d. Nerve lies above the posterior belly of digastric.

120. Complications of mumps include all except:
a. Unilateral sensorineural hearing loss.
b. Thyroiditis.
c. Pancreatitis.
d. Orchitis.
e. Palatal palsy.

121. A 55-year-old lady presented with tinnitus, dizziness and history of progressive hearing loss. Differential diagnosis includes all except:
a. Acoustic neuroma.
b. Endolymphatic hydrops.
c. Meningioma.
d. Histiocytosis X.

Answers: SECTION A

1. d	51. d	101. d
2. a	52. a	102. c
3. c	53. c	103. d
4. b	54. a	104. a
5. b	55. b	105. c
6. d	56. c	106. b
7. b	57. b	107. d
8. c	58. c	108. a
9. b	59. a	109. c
10. b	60. c	110. d
11. d	61. d	111. b
12. b	62. f	112. d
13. d	63. d	113. c
14. c	64. c	114. a
15. a	65. a	115. c
16. d	66. b	116. a
17. c	67. d	117. d
18. c	68. c	118. b
19. b	69. d	119. b
20. c	70. b	120. e
21. c	71. b	121. d
22. d	72. e	
23. c	73. b	
24. b	74. c	
25. b	75. c	
26. c	76. b	
27. a	77. b	
28. b	78. a	
29. b	79. d	
30. d	80. a	
31. d	81. b	
32. b	82. c	
33. b	83. a	
34. a	84. a	
35. e	85. b	
36. c	86. d	
37. e	87. b	
38. c	88. c	
39. c	89. b	
40. c	90. b	
41. d	91. a	
42. d	92. b	
43. c	93. c	
44. c	94. b	
45. d	95. b	
46. a	96. b	
47. c	97. c	
48. d	98. d	
49. c	99. c	
50. d	100. c	

SECTION B

1. Pinna is well formed by

    (a) 38 weeks of intra uterine life
    (b) 2 weeks of intra uterine life
    (c) 20 weeks of intra uterine life
    (d) 36 weeks of intra uterine life

2. **The length of the external auditory canal is**
    (a) 24 mm
    (b) 16 mm
    (c) 10 mm
    (d) 35 mm

3. **Shrapnel's membrane is**
    (a) Pars tensa of ear drum
    (b) Pars flaccida of ear drum
    (c) Round window
    (d) Oval window

4. **The tensor tympani muscle arises from**
    (a) Pyramidal eminence
    (b) Process cochleariformis
    (c) Bony portion of eustachean tube
    (d) Cartilagenous portion of eustachean tube

5. **The bony portion of eustachean tube is**
    (a) 36 mm
    (b) 34 mm
    (c) 24 mm
    (d) 12 mm

6. **Trautmann's triangle over lies**
    (a) Anterior cranial fossa
    (b) Posterior cranial fossa
    (c) Middle cranial fossa
    (d) Occiput

7. **Prussak's space lies between**
    (a) Neck of malleus and pars flaccida
    (b) Incus and stapes
    (c) Stapes and stapedial tendon
    (d) Lateral and superior semicircular canals

8. **Fissures of Santorini are deficiencies seen in**
    (a) Annulus of tympanic membrane
    (b) Bony portion of external ear canal
    (c) Lobule of the ear

(d) Cartilagenous portion of external ear canal

9. **The stapedius muscle arises from**
    (a) Pyramidal eminence
    (b) Eustachean tube
    (c) Processes cochleoformis
    (d) Posterior canal wall

10. **Korner's septum is**
    (a) Persistent glasserian fissure
    (b) Persistent squamo tympanic suture line
    (c) Persistent tympano mastoid suture line
    (d) Persistent petro squamous suture line

11. **Medial wall of middle ear cavity is formed by**
    (a) Tympanic membrane
    (b) Promontory
    (c) Eustachean tube
    (d) Tensor tympani muscle

12. **The semicircular canals open into the utricle by**
    (a) Two orifices
    (b) Six orifices
    (c) Three orifices
    (d) Five orifices

13. **The aditus connects**
    (a) External ear and middle ear
    (b) Middle and inner ear
    (c) Epitympanic recess to the mastoid antrum
    (d) Eustachean tube with the middle ear

14. **The pars tensa portion of tympanic membrane has**
    (a) Three layers
    (b) Two layers
    (c) Four layers
    (d) One layers

15. **Macula is found in**
    (a) Lateral semicircular canal
    (b) Posterior semicircular canal
    (c) Superior semicircular canal
    (d) Utricle and saccule

16. **The length of the eustachean tube is**

(a) 50 mm
(b) 36 mm
(c) 15 mm
(d) 10 mm

17. The normal tympanic membrane is
    (a) Yellow in colour
    (b) Pearly white in colour
    (c) Pink in colour
    (d) Red in colour

18. Supra pyramidal recess is the other name for
    (a) Superior incudal space
    (b) Cochlear recess
    (c) Facial recess
    (d) Prussak space

19. Fenestra cochlea is otherwise known as
    (a) Round window
    (b) Oval window
    (c) Eustachean tube orifice
    (d) Labyrinthine fistula

20. The round window in life is closed by
    (a) Pars flaccida
    (b) Foot plate of stapes
    (c) Tympanic membrane
    (d) Secondary tympanic membrane

21. The pyramidal eminence contains
    (a) Facial nerve
    (b) Eustachean tube
    (c) Cochlea
    (d) Stapedius muscle

22. Epitympanum is otherwise known as
    (a) Labyrinth
    (b) Middle ear proper
    (c) Attic
    (d) Cochlea

23. McEwen's triangle is a surface marking for
    (a) Mastoid antrum
    (b) Endolymphatic sac
    (c) Cochlea
    (d) Lateral semicircular canal

24. **The condyloid process of the mandible is closely related to**
    (a) Anterior wall of external auditory canal
    (b) Posterior wall of external auditory canal
    (c) Superior wall of external auditory canal
    (d) Inferior wall of external auditory canal

25. **Canal of Hugier contains**
    (a) Facial nerve
    (b) Stapedial tendon
    (c) Chorda tympani nerve
    (d) Eustachean tube

26. **The smallest ossicle in the middle ear cavity is**
    (a) The malleus
    (b) The stapes
    (c) The incus
    (d) Cochlea

27. **Fenestra vestibule is otherwise known as**
    (a) Eustachean tube orifice
    (b) Labyrinthine fistula
    (c) Round window
    (d) Oval window

28. **Ampullary crest is seen in**
    (a) Semicircular canals
    (b) Saccule
    (c) Utricle
    (d) Endolymphatic sac

29. **The inner two third of the external ear canal is formed by**
    (a) Parotid gland
    (b) Soft tissue
    (c) Bone
    (d) Cartilage

30. **Henle's spine is an important surface marking for**
    (a) Petrous apex
    (b) Mastoid antrum
    (c) Lateral semicircular canal
    (d) Lateral sinus

31. **The pinna develops from**
    (a) 1st and 2nd pharyngeal arches
    (b) 2nd and 3rd pharyngeal arches

(c) 3rd and 4th pharyngeal arches
(d) 4th and 5th pharyngeal arches

32. Perforations due to air pressure changes occur most commonly in
(a) Postero inferior quadrant of ear drum
(b) Antero inferior quadrant of ear drum
(c) Postero superior quadrant of ear drum
(d) Antero superior quadrant of ear drum

33. Which of the following gases can cause perforation of weakened ear drum?
(a) Ether
(b) Halothane
(c) Oxygen used during anaesthesia
(d) Nitrous oxide

34. The main factors causing the failure of traumatic perforation to heal on their own are
(a) Damage to the outer epithelial layer of ear drum
(b) Tissue loss and infection of the ear drum
(c) Loss of inner mucosal layer of the ear drum due to trauma
(d) Damage to the external auditory canal

35. The development of squamous epithelial cysts in the middle ear is seen following perforations of the ear drum caused by
(a) Injury to the ear drum due to sharp objects
(b) Injury to the ear drum caused by welding sparks
(c) Injury to the ear drum caused by bomb blast
(d) Injury to the ear drum due to a slap over the cheek

36. Chances of spontaneous healing of ear drum perforation is reduced in
(a) Ear drum perforations caused due to a slap over the cheek
(b) Ear drum perforations caused due to sharp objects
(c) Water sports injury
(d) Ear drum perforations caused due to sudden pressure changes during general anaesthesia

37. Battle's sign is
(a) Skin discolouration over mastoid process
(b) Reddish bulge seen over the ear drum
(c) Blueish bulge seen over the floor of the external auditory canal
(d) Linear tear of the ear drum due to injury by a sharp object

38. Battle's sign is seen in patients with
(a) Traumatic perforation of ear drum
(b) Fractures of temporal bone
(c) Blast injuries of ear drum

(d) Injuries of tympanic membrane caused by welding sparks

39. The commonest type of fracture involving the temporal bone is
(a) Longitudinal
(b) Transverse
(c) Mixed
(d) Punched out

40. Blows to temporal/ parietal areas of skull cause
(a) Transverse fracture of temporal bone
(b) Longitudinal fracture of temporal bone
(c) Mixed fracture of temporal bone
(d) Circular fracture of temporal bone

41. Inner ear is commonly involved in
(a) Longitudinal fractures of temporal bone
(b) Transverse fractures of temporal bone
(c) Circular fractures of temporal bone
(d) Fractures involving the mastoid cortex

42. Haemotympanum without bleeding from the ear is commonly seen in
(a) Transverse fractures of temporal bone
(b) Longitudinal fractures of temporal bone
(c) Circular fractures of temporal bone
(d) Punched out fractures of temporal bone

43. Secondary Endolymphatic hydrops can occur in
(a) Transverse fractures of temporal bone
(b) Longitudinal fractures of temporal bone
(c) Circular fractures of temporal bone
(d) Punched out fractures of temporal bone

44. Facial nerve injuries are common in
(a) Transverse fractures of temporal bone
(b) Longitudinal fractures of temporal bone
(c) Circular fractures of temporal bone
(d) Punched out fractures of temporal bone

45. Fluctuating deafness in a patient with temporal bone trauma is due to
(a) Injury to middle ear
(b) Injury to ear drum
(c) Perilymph fistula
(d) Injury to internal acoustic meatus

46. The edges of a traumatic perforation of ear drum is found to be everted due to
(a) Presence of adhesion

- (b) Negative pressure
- (c) Displaced ossicles
- (d) Trauma to external auditory canal

47. In transverse fracture of temporal bone, the facial nerve is injured in its
- (a) Mastoid segment
- (b) Tympanic segment
- (c) Labyrinthine segment
- (d) Intracranial segment

48. The investigation that could clinch the diagnosis of temporal bone fracture is
- (a) MRI scan
- (b) X ray temporal bones
- (c) High resolution CT scan
- (d) PET scan

49. Haematoma of auricle should be drained to prevent
- (a) Deformity of pinna
- (b) Stenosis of external auditory canal
- (c) Development of conductive deafness
- (d) Development of sensorineural hearing loss

50. The commonest cause of conductive deafness in a patient with fracture temporal bone is
- (a) Haemotympanum
- (b) Dislocation of malleus
- (c) Tympanic membrane perforation
- (d) Perilymph fistula

51. The commonest ossicular change abnormality associated with fractures of temporal bone is
- (a) Incudostapedial joint separation
- (b) Incudomalleolar joint separation
- (c) Avulsion of stapes
- (d) Incus dislocation

52. CSF otorrhoea following temporal bone fracture
- (a) Should be treated surgically
- (b) Is self-limiting in most of the cases
- (c) Should be treated by craniotomy
- (d) Can lead to fatal meningitis in all patients with temporal bone fracture

53. Severely traumatized external ear canal can cause
- (a) Conductive deafness in excess of 60db
- (b) Mixed deafness
- (c) Stenosis

(d) Brain herniation

54. Temporal bone fracture classification was first developed by
(a) Ulrich
(b) Ghorayeb
(c) Yeakley
(d) Bestle

55. Following trauma to external canal caused by fractures of temporal bone
(a) The ear must be packed to prevent bleeding
(b) The ear must be packed to prevent CSF otorrhoea
(c) The ear canal should not be packed
(d) Continuous suction should be applied to the external canal

56. Perilymph fistula should be suspected following stapedectomy
(a) If there is persistent conductive deafness following surgery
(b) Fluctuating hearing loss
(c) Absence of tinnitus
(d) Absence of vertigo

57. The aim of stapedectomy surgery in otosclerosis is
(a) To improve cochlear function
(b) To improve cochlear function by at least 50%
(c) Restoration of available cochlear function
(d) Improve cochlear function by 100%

58. Absolute contraindication for stapedectomy is
(a) Only hearing ear
(b) More than 80 dB air bone gap
(c) More than 40 dB air bone gap
(d) Negative Rinne test

59. Which of the following condition aggravate deafness due to otosclerosis
(a) Obesity
(b) Menstruation
(c) Pregnancy
(d) Menopause

60. Pure tone audiogram is a
(a) Subjective assessment of hearing levels
(b) Objective assessment of hearing levels
(c) Both subjective and objective assessment of hearing
(d) Comprehensive assessment of hearing

61. Sound inside in audiometer is generated by
(a) Equalisation circuit

(b) Interrupter switch
(c) Oscillator coil
(d) Head phones

62. Highest frequency used for bone conduction audiometry is
   (a) 12000 Hz
   (b) 10000 Hz
   (c) 4000 Hz
   (d) 1500Hz

63. Before bone conduction audiometry, masking is done
   (a) To prevent cross hearing
   (b) To diminish hearing acuity
   (c) To increase hearing acuity
   (d) To assess speech discrimination

64. Ideally air conduction audiometry should be started with
   (a) 500 Hz
   (b) 2000 Hz
   (c) 4000 Hz
   (d) 1000 Hz

65. In sensorineural hearing loss, dip will be seen in
   (a) Low frequency zone
   (b) High frequency zone
   (c) Mid frequency zone
   (d) All frequencies

66. Hearing should be tested in paediatric patients using
   (a) Tuning fork
   (b) Pure tone audiometry
   (c) Speech audiometry
   (d) Free field audiometry

67. Air conduction threshold of 90 dB and above indicates
   (a) Profound hearing loss
   (b) Mild hearing loss
   (c) Severe hearing loss
   (d) Moderate hearing loss

68. While plotting PTA values of right ear
   (a) Green ink is used
   (b) Blue ink is used
   (c) Red ink is used
   (d) Black ink is used

69. Important prerequisite for a good audiometric headphone is
   (a) It should has a flat frequency response
   (b) It should has a high frequency response
   (c) It should has a low frequency response
   (d) It should be loosely fitting

70. Cookie bite audiogram is a feature of
   (a) Noise induced hearing loss
   (b) Otosclerosis
   (c) Ossicular discontinuity
   (d) Chronic suppurative otitis media

71. Carhart's notch in a pure tone audiogram is seen in
   (a) 100 Hz range
   (b) 4000 Hz range
   (c) 1000 Hz range
   (d) 8000 Hz range

72. The presence of Carhart's notch is a feature of
   (a) Otosclerosis
   (b) Noise induced hearing loss
   (c) Congenital hearing loss
   (d) Impacted cerumen

73. Presence of high frequency sensorineural hearing loss is a feature of
   (a) Impacted wax
   (b) Chronic suppurative otitis media
   (c) Noised induced hearing loss
   (d) Meniere's disease

74. In PTA the sound produced by the audiometer is
   (a) Continuous
   (b) Interrupted
   (c) A musical note
   (d) A word

75. Weber's test assesses
   (a) Air condition threshold
   (b) Bone conduction threshold
   (c) Inter aural sound attenuation
   (d) Speech threshold

76. Human ears are most sensitive around
   (a) 4000 Hz frequency range
   (b) 2000 Hz frequency range
   (c) 100 Hz frequency range

(d) 6000 Hz frequency range

77. Type A tympanometric curve suggests
   (a) Conductive deafness
   (b) Retro cochlear deafness
   (c) Otosclerosis
   (d) Normal middle ear function

78. Type Ad tympanometric curve suggests
   (a) Ossicular discontinuity
   (b) Chronic suppurative otitis media
   (c) Otosclerosis
   (d) Normal middle ear function

79. Type As tympanometric curve suggests
   (a) Ossicular discontinuity
   (b) Chronic suppurative otitis media
   (c) Otosclerosis
   (d) Normal middle ear function

80. Faulty position of ear phones in PTA causes
   (a) 60 dB threshold variation
   (b) 15 dB threshold variation
   (c) 80 dB threshold variation
   (d) 5 dB threshold variation

81. Stenger's test is used to
   (a) Identify conductive deafness
   (b) Identify malingering
   (c) Identify sensorineural hearing loss
   (d) Quantify conductive deafness

82. In PTA to illustrate recordings from left ear
   (a) Blue colour is used
   (b) Red colour is used
   (c) Black colour is used
   (d) Green colour is used

83. Salicylate induced tinnitus is caused by
   (a) Increased intracellular calcium in OHC
   (b) Decreased intracellular sodium in OHC
   (c) Increased intracellular potassium in OHC
   (d) Decreased intracellular potassium in OHC

84. Tinnitus retraining therapy is based on
   (a) Habituation

(b) Improving blood supply to inner ear
(c) Administration of neurotropic vitamins
(d) Administration of calcium

85. Stress aggravates tinnitus by
(a) Acting on the inner hair cells
(b) Acting on the hearing centres of brain
(c) Acting on the auditory nerves
(d) Acting on lateral olivocochlear system

86. Auditory hallucinations are generated in
(a) Inner ear
(b) Middle ear
(c) Auditory nerve
(d) Cortex

87. Tinnitus makers should be used for at least
(a) Half hour a day
(b) 6-8 hours a day
(c) 2 hours a day
(d) 3 hours a day

88. The characteristic feature of objective tinnitus is
(a) It is heard only by the patient
(b) It is heard by the observer and patient
(c) It is meaningful words heard by the patient
(d) It is roaring in nature

89. The characteristic feature of subjective tinnitus is
(a) It is heard only by the patient
(b) It is heard by the observer and patient
(c) It is meaningful words heard by the patient
(d) It is roaring in nature

90. High frequency tinnitus is seen in
(a) Noise induced hearing loss
(b) Presbyacusis
(c) Meniere's disease
(d) Adhesive otitis media

91. Low frequency tinnitus is seen in
(a) Noise induced hearing loss
(b) Presbyacusis
(c) Meniere's disease
(d) Adhesive otitis media

92. Subjective tinnitus is otherwise known as
    (a) Tinnitus aurium
    (b) Auditory hallucination
    (c) Vascular sound
    (d) Patulous eustachean tube

93. The most common cause of pulsatile venous tinnitus in obese female patients is
    (a) Meniere's disease
    (b) Vestibular schwannoma
    (c) Pseudotumor cerebri syndrome
    (d) High jugular bulb

94. The most accepted pathophysiology of tinnitus is
    (a) Damage to middle ear
    (b) Damage to outer hair cell
    (c) Damage to auditory nerve
    (d) Damage to brain stem

95. The feature of in active mucosal chronic otitis media is
    (a) Normal ear drum
    (b) Middle ear is inflamed
    (c) Mastoid tip cells are inflamed
    (d) Middle ear mucosa and mastoid cells are normal

96. Perforations in tubotympanic type of ear disease is
    (a) Round in shape
    (b) Spherical in shape
    (c) Reniform in shape
    (d) Stellate shape

97. Fistula test is positive in
    (a) Acute mastoiditis
    (b) Acute petrositis
    (c) Erosion of lateral canal
    (d) Erosion of basal turn of cochlea

98. Commonest organism isolated from lateral sinus thrombophlebitis in prebiotic era was
    (a) Pseudomonas
    (b) Anaerobes
    (c) Staphylococci
    (d) Beta haemolytic streptococci

99. Acute necrotizing otitis media can lead to
    (a) Secondary acquired cholesteatoma
    (b) Primary acquired cholesteatoma

(c) Congenital cholesteatoma
(d) Labyrinthitis granuloma

100. The difference between subtotal perforation and total perforation is
    (a) Involvement of attic in total perforation
    (b) Sparing of annulus in total perforation
    (c) Destruction of annulus in total perforation
    (d) Involvement of ossicles in subtotal perforation

101. Pain in the ear in a patient with tubotympanic disease is due to
    (a) Otitis externa
    (b) Malignant otitis externa
    (c) Labyrinthitis
    (d) Lateral sinus thrombophlebitis

102. Major organisms seen in discharge from chronic suppurative otitis media are
    (a) Mostly gram positive organisms
    (b) Mostly gram negative organisms
    (c) Viruses
    (d) Fungi

103. Symptomatic triad of acute mastoiditis are
    (a) Otalgia, post auricular pain, giddiness
    (b) Otalgia, post auricular pain, fever
    (c) Otalgia, post auricular pain, vomiting
    (d) Otalgia, CSF otorrhoea, giddiness

104. Gradenigo syndrome is
    (a) Acute mastoiditis
    (b) Acute petrositis
    (c) Lateral sinus thrombosis
    (d) Labyrinthitis

105. Attico antral ear disease is characterised by
    (a) Profuse discharge
    (b) Serosanguinous discharge
    (c) Mucoid discharge
    (d) Scanty discharge

106. The feature of inactive mucosal chronic otitis media is
    (a) Normal ear drum
    (b) Middle ear is inflamed
    (c) Mastoid tip cells are inflamed
    (d) Middle ear mucosa and mastoid cells are normal

107. Myringoplasty is

(a) Reconstruction of ear drum only
(b) Reconstruction of ear drum and ossicles
(c) Reconstruction of ossicles alone
(d) Reconstruction of middle ear ossicles with mastoidectomy

108. Dimeric ear drum is seen in
    (a) Healed CSOM
    (b) Attico antral disease
    (c) ASOM
    (d) Adhesive otitis media

109. Cawthorne theory of cholesteatoma genesis states that
    (a) Cholesteatoma arises due to tubal block
    (b) It arises from embryonic cell rests
    (c) It arises due to basal cell hyperplasia
    (d) It arises due to invagination of pars flaccida

110. Hearing loss in safe type of CSOM is commonly
    (a) Conductive in nature
    (b) Sensorineural in nature
    (c) Mixed in nature
    (d) Normal hearing

111. Hearing loss in safe type of CSOM is commonly
    (a) Between 30-40 dB
    (b) Above 60 dB
    (c) Above 80 dB
    (d) Total hearing loss

112. Odour of cholesteatoma discharge is
    (a) Fruity
    (b) Musty
    (c) Rotten egg
    (d) Odourless

113. Which is not a predisposing factor for development of Meniere's disease
    (a) Fibrosis of sac
    (b) Inner ear viral infection
    (c) Altered glycoprotein metabolism
    (d) Pneumatized periaqueductal region

114. Viruses that could cause Meniere's disease commonly belong to
    (a) Rhinovirus group
    (b) Enterovirus group
    (c) Neurotropic group
    (d) Polio virus

115. Which of the following could be the possible anatomical cause for Meniere's disease
    (a) Smaller vestibular aqueduct
    (b) Large vestibular aqueduct
    (c) Enlarged basal turn of cochlea
    (d) Fixed foot plate (congenital)

116. Hearing loss in Meniere's patient involves
    (a) Low frequency
    (b) Mid frequency
    (c) High frequency
    (d) All frequency ranges

117. The osmolality of endolymph
    (a) Increases from apex to the base of cochlea
    (b) Decreases from apex to the base of cochlea
    (c) Is the same throughout the labyrinth
    (d) Is the most in the semicircular canals

118. Portmann's operation in the management of Meniere's disease is
    (a) Cortical mastoidectomy
    (b) Labyrinthectomy
    (c) Endolymphatic sac decompression
    (d) Grommet insertion

119. Labyrinthectomy is indicated treatment modality in
    (a) Patients with acute Meniere's disease
    (b) Patients with Tumarkin's crisis
    (c) Patients with Lermoyez syndrome
    (d) Meniere's disease with severe hearing loss

120. Groningen criteria for the diagnosis of Meniere's is
    (a) Deafness should be sensorineural alone
    (b) Deafness should be conductive alone
    (c) Deafness should be mixed
    (d) Total deafness

121. Which is the contraindication of vibrator therapy in Meniere's disease?
    (a) Acute vomiting
    (b) Perilymph fistula
    (c) Giddiness
    (d) Presence of nystagmus

122. Trauma causes Meniere's disease by
    (a) Increasing endolymph secretion

    (b) Releasing debris into endolymph
    (c) Causing damage to ear drum
    (d) Causing damage to round window

123. **Normal summating potential : action potential is**
    (a) 1 : 8
    (b) 2 : 8
    (c) 1 : 3
    (d) 1 : 1

124. **Pars inferior portion of membranous labyrinth includes**
    (a) Cochlea duct and saccule
    (b) Utricle
    (c) Semicircular canal
    (d) Ampulla

125. **ECOG findings in Meniere's disease include**
    (a) Widened summating potential action potential complex
    (b) Narrow action potential
    (c) Negative potential
    (d) Normal study

126. **Lawrence hypothesis of Endolymphatic circulation says**
    (a) The fluid circulates radially
    (b) The fluid circulates axially
    (c) The fluid circulates longitudinally
    (d) Fluid circulates both radially and longitudinally

127. **In Tumarkin's crisis a patient**
    (a) Has vertigo (central)
    (b) Has peripheral type of vertigo
    (c) Has drop attacks and loss of consciousness
    (d) Has tinnitus alone

128. **Chronic suppurative otitis media (CSOM) causes secondary Meniere's disease due to**
    (a) Percolation of toxins to inner ear
    (b) Damage to ossicles
    (c) Damage to basal turn of cochlea
    (d) Damage to Endolymphatic sac

129. **The feature of cochlear Meniere's include**
    (a) Fluctuating hearing loss alone
    (b) Vertigo alone

(c) Hearing loss improves when giddiness sets in
(d) Drop attacks

130. In early stages of Meniere's disease
    (a) The whole membranous labyrinth is distended
    (b) Pars superior portion is distended
    (c) Pars inferior portion is distended
    (d) Lateral canal is distended

131. Diazepam when administered to a patient with Meniere's disease act by
    (a) Its action on ACE inhibitors
    (b) Stimulating cerebellar GABAergic neurons
    (c) Depressing cerebellar GABAergic neurons
    (d) Increases diuresis

132. Furstenberg diet is
    (a) Low fat diet
    (b) Salt free diet
    (c) Sugar free diet
    (d) Diet mixed with honey

133. Anatomical landmark for Endolymphatic sac is
    (a) Facial nerve
    (b) Lateral semicircular canal
    (c) Basal turn of cochlea
    (d) Donaldson's line

134. Which of the following condition could cause secondary Meniere's disease?
    (a) Syphilis
    (b) Leprosy
    (c) Tuberculosis
    (d) Presbyacusis

135. Aural fullness in Meniere's disease is caused by
    (a) Enlarging membranous labyrinth
    (b) Enlarged sac alone
    (c) Enlarged utricle alone
    (d) Enlarged lateral semicircular canal alone

136. Among these tests which is diagnostic in Meniere's disease
    (a) Tuning fork test
    (b) Electrocochleography
    (c) PTA
    (d) ENG

137. The angulation of eustachean tube in an adult is

(a) 45 degrees
(b) 10 degrees
(c) 25 degrees
(d) 160 degrees

138. In infants the inclination of eustachean tube is
    (a) 45 degrees
    (b) 10 degrees
    (c) 25 degrees
    (d) 160 degrees

139. Length of Eustachian tube in adult is
    (a) 100 mm
    (b) 38 mm
    (c) 15 mm
    (d) 18 mm

140. Protympanum is
    (a) Cartilagenous portion of ET
    (b) Terminal end of ET
    (c) Bony portion of ET
    (d) Torus tubaris

141. The shape of the lumen of osseous portion of ET is
    (a) Circular
    (b) Oval
    (c) Triangular
    (d) Slit like

142. During Valsalva manoeuvre
    (a) Bony portion of ET opens
    (b) Hypo tympanic end of ET opens
    (c) Cartilagenous portion opens
    (d) Tubal end closes

143. Which of the following statement is correct?
    (a) Anterior 1/3 of ET is bony
    (b) Anterior 2/3 of ET is bony
    (c) Anterior 1/3 is Cartilagenous
    (d) Posterior 1/3 is bony

144. The angle between the bony and cartilagenous portions of ET is
    (a) 160 degrees
    (b) 70 degrees
    (c) 90 degrees
    (d) 100 degrees

145. Active dilatation of ET is caused by
    (a) Contraction of tensor veli palatine
    (b) Contraction of levator veli palatine
    (c) Contraction of salphigopharyngeus
    (d) Contraction of palatoglossus

146. Cartilagenous portion of ET is deficient
    (a) Superiorly
    (b) Laterally
    (c) Inferolaterally
    (d) Superolaterally

147. Protympanum lies completely within
    (a) Tympanic portion of temporal bone
    (b) Mastoid portion of temporal bone
    (c) Petrous portion of temporal bone
    (d) Squamous portion of temporal bone

148. Mucous glands predominate in
    (a) Tympanic end of ET
    (b) Protympanum
    (c) Bony portion of temporal bone
    (d) Nasopharyngeal orifice of ET

149. Sonotubometry is used to
    (a) Assess middle ear function
    (b) Assess ET function
    (c) Identifying autophony
    (d) Identifying sensorineural hearing loss

150. The sound frequency used in Sonotubometry is
    (a) 8000 Hz
    (b) 4000 Hz
    (c) 10 000 Hz
    (d) 100 Hz

151. Man in barrel sensation is caused by
    (a) ET block
    (b) Patulous ET
    (c) Eustachean cattarl
    (d) Tubal tonsil enlargement

152. Palatal myoclonus causes
    (a) Clicking sound in the ear
    (b) Ear block

(c) Subjective tinnitus
(d) Eustachean catarrh

153. Narrowest potion of ET is seen in
    (a) Its pharyngeal end
    (b) Hypo tympanum
    (c) Junction of bony and cartilagenous portions
    (d) Middle of bony portion

154. Cartilage of ET is shaped like a
    (a) Cylinder
    (b) Cone
    (c) Shepard's crook
    (d) Pyramidal

155. Lymphoid tissue surrounding the ET opening in nasopharynx is known as
    (a) Adenoid
    (b) Gerlat's tonsil
    (c) Lingual tonsil
    (d) Palatine tonsil

156. Temporary ET dysfunction is an indication for
    (a) Myringotomy
    (b) Grommet insertion
    (c) Cortical mastoidectomy
    (d) Myringoplasty

157. The number of muscles associated with ET is
    (a) 6
    (b) 2
    (c) 4
    (d) 1

158. Mucosa lining the ET is
    (a) Ciliated columnar
    (b) Cuboidal
    (c) Pavement
    (d) Squamous

159. Cholesteatoma sac contains
    (a) Mucoid materials
    (b) Desquamated squamous epithelium
    (c) Cuboidal epithelium
    (d) Cholesterol crystals

160. Cholesteatoma is defined as skin in wrong place because

(a) Of accumulation of keratin
(b) Of accumulation of sebaceous glands
(c) Of accumulation of sweat glands
(d) Of accumulation of cholesterol

161. The layer of cholesteatoma in direct contact with bone is
    (a) Matrix
    (b) Cyst wall
    (c) Perimatrix
    (d) Cuboidal cell layer

162. Perimatrix layer of cholesteatoma contains
    (a) Squamous epithelium
    (b) Keratinous layer
    (c) Granulation tissue
    (d) Cuboidal epithelium

163. Toss theory of cholesteatoma postulates that
    (a) It could be caused by attic retraction
    (b) Due to congenital epithelial cell rest
    (c) It could be due to metaplasia
    (d) Due to epithelial migration through attic perforation

164. Commonly attic cholesteatoma starts from
    (a) Prussak's space
    (b) Superior incudal space
    (c) Posterior incudal space
    (d) Facial recess

165. Secondary acquired cholesteatoma is caused by
    (a) Attic retraction
    (b) Acute necrotizing otitis media
    (c) Secretory otitis media
    (d) Eustachean tube blockage

166. Classic features of acute necrotizing otitis media is
    (a) Later perforation of ear drum
    (b) Mucoid secretion
    (c) Foul smelling aural secretion
    (d) Mild hearing loss

167. Prussak's space is bounded superiorly by
    (a) Lateral malleolar fold
    (b) Medial malleolar fold
    (c) Posterior malleolar fold
    (d) Anterior malleolar fold

168. In acute necrotizing otitis media
    (a) Pars tensa alone is destroyed
    (b) Handle of malleolus alone is destroyed
    (c) Tympanic membrane along with annulus is destroyed
    (d) Incus alone is destroyed

169. In bridging cholesteatoma
    (a) Hearing is normal
    (b) There is sensory neural hearing loss
    (c) There is mixed hearing loss
    (d) There is severe conductive hearing loss

170. Teel's epithelial cell rest theory is used to explain
    (a) Primary acquired cholesteatoma
    (b) Secondary acquired cholesteatoma
    (c) Congenital cholesteatoma
    (d) Acute necrotizing otitis media

171. Pressure induced bone necrosis in cholesteatoma is caused by
    (a) Activation of osteoclasts
    (b) Hyperaemic decalcification
    (c) Activation of osteoblasts
    (d) Infection

172. CT scan is indicated in a patient with cholesteatoma
    (a) To rule out external canal involvement
    (b) To look for intracranial complications
    (c) To access the integrity of ossicular chain
    (d) To look for round window reflex

173. The role of pneumatic otoscopy in a patient with cholesteatoma is
    (a) To assess the size of perforation
    (b) To rule out intracranial complications
    (c) To perform fistula test
    (d) To assess patient's hearing level

174. Which of the following structures get commonly eroded in cholesteatoma
    (a) Head of malleus
    (b) Handle of malleus
    (c) Foot plate
    (d) Long process of incus

175. The absolute indication of canal wall down mastoidectomy is
    (a) Erosion of posterior canal wall by cholesteatoma
    (b) Tubotympanic ear disease
    (c) Meniere's disease
    (d) CSF otorrhoea

176. Surface marking for mastoid antrum is
    (a) Lobule of ear
    (b) McEwen's triangle
    (c) Antihelix
    (d) Helix

ANSWERS: SECTION B

1. (c)
2. (a)
3. (b)
4. (d)
5. (d)
6. (b)
7. (a)
8. (d)
9. (a)
10. (d)
11. (b)
12. (d)
13. (c)
14. (a)
15. (d)
16. (b)
17. (b)
18. (c)
19. (a)
20. (d)
21. (d)
22. (c)
23. (a)
24. (a)
25. (c)
26. (b)
27. (d)
28. (a)
29. (c)
30. (b)
31. (a)
32. (b)
33. (d)
34. (b)
35. (c)
36. (c)
37. (a)
38. (b)
39. (a)
40. (b)
41. (b)

42. (a)
43. (a)
44. (a)
45. (c)
46. (b)
47. (c)
48. (c)
49. (a)
50. (a)
51. (a)
52. (b)
53. (c)
54. (a)
55. (c)
56. (b)
57. (c)
58. (a)
59. (c)
60. (a)
61. (c)
62. (c)
63. (a)
64. (d)
65. (b)
66. (d)
67. (a)
68. (c)
69. (a)
70. (b)
71. (b)
72. (a)
73. (c)
74. (b)
75. (c)
76. (b)
77. (d)
78. (a)
79. (c)
80. (b)
81. (b)
82. (a)
83. (c)
84. (a)
85. (d)
86. (d)
87. (b)

88. (b)
89. (a)
90. (c)
91. (a)
92. (c)
93. (b)
94. (d)
95. (c)
96. (c)
97. (d)
98. (a)
99. (a)
100. (c)
101. (a)
102. (b)
103. (b)
104. (b)
105. (d)
106. (d)
107. (a)
108. (d)
109. (a)
110. (a)
111. (c)
112. (b)
113. (d)
114. (c)
115. (a)
116. (a)
117. (a)
118. (c)
119. (d)
120. (a)
121. (b)
122. (b)
123. (c)
124. (a)
125. (a)
126. (d)
127. (c)
128. (a)
129. (a)
130. (c)
131. (b)
132. (b)
133. (d)

134.	(a)
135.	(a)
136.	(b)
137.	(a)
138.	(b)
139.	(b)
140.	(c)
141.	(c)
142.	(c)
143.	(d)
144.	(a)
145.	(a)
146.	(c)
147.	(c)
148.	(d)
149.	(b)
150.	(a)
151.	(b)
152.	(a)
153.	(c)
154.	(c)
155.	(b)
156.	(b)
157.	(c)
158.	(a)
159.	(b)
160.	(a)
161.	(c)
162.	(a)
163.	(a)
164.	(a)
165.	(b)
166.	(c)
167.	(a)
168.	(c)
169.	(a)
170.	(c)
171.	(b)
172.	(b)
173.	(c)
174.	(d)
175.	(a)
176.	(b)

www.ingramcontent.com/pod-product-compliance
Lightning Source LLC
Chambersburg PA
CBHW051055180526
45172CB00002B/651